How to Study and Master Any Subject - *Quickly!*

A College Professor Reveals 8 Fast Learning Methods That Really Work!

Mario J. Giordano

Published by *G.E.T. Management, LLC*

U.S.A.

Copyright © 2016 by G.E.T. Management, LLC.

All rights reserved. Compiled in the United States of America. No part of this book may be used or reproduced in any manner whatsoever without written permission except in the case of brief quotations embodied in critical articles or reviews.

ISBN-13: 978-1532989940
ISBN-10: 1532989946

Forward

The first edition of this book was written and published by Prof. Giordano in 1975 under the title," *Basic Learning Secrets That Pay Off*". As such, you will find some temporal references that may seem dated, such as the inability to bring a computer into the classroom in FLM #4. This isn't such an odd statement, considering that when Prof. Giordano wrote this book, the computer he was programming was three-stories high and required a dedicated air-conditioning system to keep from overheating. We have left the text as it was originally written to remain faithful to the author's intent and are sure that the concepts discussed are just as valid today as they were in the past. My brothers, Edmund F. Giordano, Dr. Gary F. Giordano and I are proud and happy to share a small part of our father's legacy with those who value, as much as we do, the importance of an education and self-improvement. *– Dr. Thomas V. Giordano*

TABLE OF CONTENTS

INTRODUCTION	ii
WHAT YOU WILL GET FROM THIS REPORT	ii
WHY SHOULD YOU LEARN HOW TO LEARN?	iii
HOW TO MAKE LEARNING DIFFICULT	iv
FLM #1: THE THREE GOLDEN RULES OF LEARNING	1
FLM #2: A FAST STUDY METHOD THAT GUARANTEES HIGH TEST SCORES	9
FLM #3: SPEED LEARNING THROUGH INDIVIDUALIZED INSTRUCTION	15
FLM #4: UNDERSTANDING BY DEMONSTRATING WITH OBJECTS	21
FLM #5: FAST LEARNING BY REMOVING UNIMPORTANT DATA	25
FLM #6: FLASH READING FOR UNDERSTANDING	27
FLM #7: MINI-COURSES FROM YOUR DICTIONARY	31
FLM #8: TRICKS TO MEMORIZING: IT'S EASY WHEN YOU KNOW HOW	37
SOME LAST WORDS	43
ABOUT THE AUTHOR	45

INTRODUCTION

Let's first set the tone for this report. The one thing I want to do, above all, is give you this important information in the simplest, friendliest way I can. So, from this point forward, think of me as a friend who is sharing with you what he has learned about learning.

As you study this report, picture yourself just having a conversation with a friend. Don't look for catchy phrases, picturesque writing or grammatically perfect prose. It's only the information I want you to have. Information that will become an important tool for your survival in the years to come.

WHAT YOU WILL GET FROM THIS REPORT

I know this report will change your life for the better. That's why I feel very good about getting it to you. It has changed my life and those of hundreds of others who now know the same information, it all has to do with knowing how you can learn any body of knowledge quickly and thoroughly, even if you never had success at learning before. It also has to do with saying "bunk" to those who have said that knowing how to learn is for those with a high IQ. I am here to tell you, and I hope to convince you, that you no longer have to believe that nonsense. Learning ability and skills are not for the selected few, only. In fact, I have conclusive proof that 95% of our population could learn anything, given enough time. This means that the only difference between you and a genius is the length of time you both need to master a subject. If you can find a way to shorten that length of time, you will have moved closer to the genius level.

This report is *THE WAY*. It contains eight fast-learning methods (*FLMS*) that will make you a much faster learner. By the time you finish this report, you will know:

1. How to remove the one major barrier to understanding.

2. How to quickly absorb the basics of any subject and give yourself a bedrock foundation to what you want to know.

3. How to make it almost impossible for anyone (even a teacher) to ask you a question you cannot answer correctly.

4. How to learn on your own (without classes and teachers) through a fool-proof method that has been suppressed by educators for years.

5. How to quickly absorb and understand whole books.

6. How to "*lay in concrete*" a full understanding of the subject you are studying through the use of simple bric-a-brac found in any home.

Mario J. Giordano

7. How to learn the secrets of acquiring quick understanding through an almost unknown use of the dictionary.

8. How to burn whole lists of data into your memory so that you can automatically recall them anytime.

WHY SHOULD YOU LEARN HOW TO LEARN?

Most skills depend upon three primary abilities: to read with understanding; to write clearly; and to calculate accurately. Abilities in these areas are necessary for advancement in any field. But, believe it or not, these are not the basics of learning. Before you can master reading, writing and arithmetic, you must first learn how to learn.

Yes, "*learning*" is a skill that must be learned. It does not come automatically. And, strangely enough, it is not taught in school!

Now, I've been an educator for over two decades. In all that time, I've never seen a course designed that effectively taught people how to learn. And that skill is more important today than in any time in the past!

To survive these days, you had better know how to learn, quickly. You can no longer get away with being like the unschooled mechanic who spent 20 years at his trade and thinks he knows all he needs to know about mechanics. Believe me, he doesn't. Most of what he learned, he learned by trial and error. He rarely knows *WHY* things are the way they are. That's the difference between a mechanic and an engineer. The engineer knows how *and* why. This is also the difference between a small income and a large one.

So, why should you learn how to learn? To survive better, that's why! If you cannot learn, you cannot find out how "to do." And, if you can't "do" you'll have a difficult time getting along in this highly technical age we live in.

HOW TO MAKE LEARNING DIFFICULT

Before you attempt to learn another thing, let me tell you why many find learning so difficult. It starts with four basic mistakes people make when they first decide to learn a body of knowledge. Let's take them one at a time.

First, some of us start with the wrong attitude. It is a peculiar thing that, when a person enters the study of a subject he already knows *something* about, he adopts the attitude (mostly without his knowing it) that he already knows the data. This attitude of "*knowing it all already*" is a common blockage to learning. The worst thing about it is that is never allows the student to really dig into the data. Also, he never really learns how to use the material. The result is that the learner becomes, at best, a person who knows only the "*buzz*" words. He never quite masters the subject.

How to Study and Master Any Subject – Quickly!

When you start reading the material in the pages that follow, please don't adopt the attitude that you have already heard it before, that you already know much of what I'm going to say. Rather, assume the innocence of a child discovering something new. This approach helps you get all the benefits.

A second reason why learning can be difficult is because learning deals mostly with symbols. We know them as words and numbers. They represent the objects and abstract concepts of life.

For instance, the word "tree" is a symbol for the real thing. In learning, we rarely deal with trees themselves but with the symbol that stands for "tree." That's when we run into trouble. A symbol is bound to mean different things to different people because of different points of view. *Teaching* may be the *same* for everyone in a classroom, but learning is *different* for each person there.

So, another reason why learning fails, when it fails, is mostly because teaching is mostly done through symbols and not with the objects they represent.

A third reason why learning is so difficult for many is because *understanding* data and *applying* data learned are *two different things*. If you dealt with the actual mass or object as you were learning - using immediately the things you've learned - you would not only understand the material better, but you would also *know how to use it*.

The Iranians say that knowledge is power. The ability to use what you know, however, is even more powerful.

In learning the Fast Learning Methods (*FLM*s) in this report, continually ask yourself, "How can I use this data?" or "How is this information being used already by others?" Then, try to put these FLMs to immediate use. When you do this, the facts become *working* tools that increase your ability to survive in the world of work.

Fourthly, being unable to concentrate attention, really not *intending* to learn, is also a barrier to learning.

So, give these pages the closest attention you have ever given anything. Really *INTEND* to learn the data described here. Don't give it just a quick reading. Instead, really concentrate on what it says.

Success in life depends on squarely facing it and carrying all actions to a conclusion. So, apply your *undivided attention* and *honest intention* to the study of this report.

In summary, and before you continue, do these things:

- Assume that you never heard anything about the material that follows;
- Mentally picture the object and experiences that are symbolized in the words that follow, imagine how the facts can be used, and immediately use them, and;

- Really intend that you are going to get the most from this report.

If you do these things, you can't lose!

FAST LEARNING METHOD #1

THE THREE GOLDEN RULES OF LEARNING

AFTER YOU HAVE STUDIED AND LEARNED THIS FLM, YOU WILL HAVE REMOVED THE BIGGEST BARRIER TO UNDERSTANDING.

I'm happy to say that the vast majority of the thousands of students who passed through my classes pass my courses. But, even though I did my best to help the marginal students, some of them managed to fail. These flunks always left me with a sense of failure, too. So, I decided long ago to find the answer to this problem. What did these failing students have in common that made them fail? What teaching technique would make sure that even the worst students would pass my courses?

I started my search by reading books written by fellow educators. Some claimed that "proper motivation" was the key; others stated that no one could successfully teach past a low I.Q., and it was useless to try. I came across at least three or four more "logical" answers. Somehow, they never quite satisfied me. None of the answers proved to be the common denominator of why people fail to learn.

The first hint of such a thing came from the writings of L. Ron Hubbard, the founder of Scientology. He, too, had the same problem: people failing to learn in his training courses. He, too, decided to find out why.

Some of what he discovered, plus some data that I picked up elsewhere, have been combined to form this "Fast Learning Method" (FLM). It is so simple that most people, hearing it for the first time, can't believe it works as well as it does. Don't let this influence you, though.

Believe me, *this is the first and basic reason why people fail to learn.*

The best way to understand this reason is to look at the anatomy of failure in reverse - what its makeup is - starting with the last action of a failing student to the very first action that made failure a sure thing. It goes something like this:

To get to the last action (final failure or dropping out) a person first fails tests. But, before that, he arrives at a point where he does not understand the data of the subject. Even before that point, though - *and this is where the key of this FLM is found* - he consistently makes the one basic error that failing students almost always make: *HE DOES NOT* go through the trouble of defining the words he didn't understand in his study of the subject, especially the special terms.

We need go no further. The beginning of failure *IS THE UNDEFINED WORD.*

The first action that leads to failure-to-learn, then, is to skip over words you do not understand.

Now, I know this sounds too simple to be true. Being human, we are inclined to disregard simple explanations. We seem to think that an answer has to be complex to be correct. But, extensive investigation

How to Study and Master Any Subject – Quickly!

by L. Ron Hubbard and somewhat by me reveals that the basic answer to most complex problems is *usually* very simple, not complex. The same holds true for the answer to why people fail to learn.

The common denominator of almost all failure-to-learn is the misunderstood - or not understood - word (nomenclature].

THE GREATEST BARRIER TO LEARNING

Nomenclature, then - the terms used to describe a body of knowledge - *is* the greatest barrier to learning. When you do *not* know the meanings of the words in a subject (the word "grammar" for instance), you cannot use the data to reach your goals. Since subject areas are as valuable to the extent that they can be used, unlearned subjects are useless.

Before you can understand a subject, before you can use it or communicate it to others, you must know, accurately, all the special terms used in it. The reason is fairly simple: without an exact meaning for each word, the subject becomes - to varying degrees - a *confusion*. And, this confusion begins to be felt after the *first* "not-known word" is skipped over.

As a teacher, in both high school and college, I've observed hundreds of students trying to learn a subject without taking the time to understand the words of that subject. Confusion is always the result, sometimes very early. And whenever I was able to convince a student that he must learn the language of that subject, miraculous changes for the better took place soon after.

I know without doubt *that the only reason a person can't understand or finish a subject is because he has not bothered to learn the accurate definitions and meanings of all the special words of that subject.*

So, the basic barrier to learning turns out to be quite simple: not knowing the nomenclature, not knowing the meanings of words.

When you go past words that you don't understand, you are dooming yourself to failure in that subject. Upon those words – and the meanings of those words - rests the *understanding* of more advanced data in that subject. If you are to know the *advanced* data, you must build that advanced data on a solid understanding of basic nomenclature.

I have thoroughly tested this out, as have others. I found that, when a student is in a state of confusion about his studies, it is *always* because he has gone past words he doesn't understand.

Words with no meanings - and even the partially understood words - cause confusion and failure. Put in another way, undefined words cause unaligned data. They float in limbo, so to speak. And, the result is confusion. This causes an inability to understand the subject, which results in failure to use that body of knowledge for your own gain.

Mario J. Giordano

For example, have you ever come to the end of a page and not remembered what you read? We all have; but did you ever try to find out why? If you test yourself with the secret you've just learned, you'll find that somewhere on that page you were in *full* understanding before you went into a dullness. Just *before* that dullness is a word you did not understand and *bypassed*. Look up that word; learn its meaning; use it in a few sentences and you become magically awake again.

Here is another example: suppose I said a man was suffering from a myocardial infarction and because of this, he was laid-up for two months. If you didn't know the exact meaning of myocardial infarction, you would never get a full understanding of what was wrong with the person, even if you were a doctor who assumed he knew!! There would be a sense of confusion about the entire statement and condition.

But, if you then found that myocardial infarction had to do with a blockage of blood vessels that feed heart muscles - and thus caused a heart attack - you would understand what physically happened to the person.

So, make no mistake about this. It's the "not-understood" and "misunderstood words" you leave undefined that cause your *main* problems in learning. That's a big statement, but it's true.

THE FIRST GOLDEN RULE OF LEARNING

So, let me repeat what really turns out to be the basic rule for learning anything:

NEVER GO PAST WORDS YOU CANNOT DEFINE WITHOUT HESITATION.

    NEVER GO PAST WORDS YOU CANNOT DEFINE WITHOUT HESITATION.

        NEVER GO PAST WORDS YOU CANNOT DEFINE WITHOUT HESITATION.

            NEVER GO PAST WORDS YOU CANNOT DEFINE WITHOUT HESITATION.

        NEVER GO PAST WORDS YOU CANNOT DEFINE WITHOUT HESITATION.

    NEVER GO PAST WORDS YOU CANNOT DEFINE WITHOUT HESITATION.

NEVER GO PAST WORDS YOU CANNOT DEFINE WITHOUT HESITATION.

WHAT HAPPENS WHEN YOU IGNORE THE FIRST GOLDEN RULE OF LEARNING?

With this Golden Rule, we are looking at the very basic truth in learning. Just think for a minute what it means to read, write, or think in words not understood or are merely fuzzy in your understanding. Now, think, too, about trying to learn a subject but refusing (or neglecting) to look up the meanings of words used to describe the subject. How much success do you think you will have in trying to apply what you have learned? Failure is the certain outcome. Or, at best, just getting by.

Failure starts at the very first new word in a subject that is skipped over without defining. This is the start of a down-spiraling in understanding that soon leads to failure. Let's look a little closer to see how this works.

Picture a student starting the study of accounting; he opens the book to *Chapter One* because the next day's lesson is based on it. As he reads along, he comes to the technical word, "assets." Now, most beginning students do not know the definition of "asset" or have some fuzzy idea of what it means. (The word merely means "things owned.")

Also, let's assume, real or not, that we all have a *certain amount of attention*; and, that it can be broken up into a number of attention parts. Finally, assume that attention parts will stick to "*not know*" mysteries.

I use this analogy because it describes so well what happens when we continue to skip over words we do not understand. Now, let's get back to our student who is studying accounting.

As he reads, he comes across the new word, "assets." He does not define it. Several attention parts stick to that undefined word while the student reads on. He now has subtracted some attention from what he had available and actually proceeds in his study with less awareness and less ability. Some of his attention is actually stuck back on that undefined word.

Further on down the page he comes to the phrase, "*Accounts Receivable*." The author says, "this is an asset." It is easy to see what follows: the student can't grasp the full meaning of "Accounts Receivable" because he has never fully defined the word "asset."

From here on, the student begins to develop a growing confusion around each undefined word, and a *further loss of attention parts*. The more attention lost through undefined words, the less attention the student has available for study. And so it goes.

This process, once started, can only get worse. More words are missed. More data are thrown into confusion. More attention is lost to confusion. Failure results.

I've observed hundreds of students go through this route after ignoring the first Golden Rule of Learning. They actually go through physical changes, too. This is what physically happens, step-by-step.

1. At the end of the page, he gets the feeling of not-knowing what he read - a blank feeling. He gets a blank look on his face.

2. At the end of several pages of study, he begins yawning. And well he should since he has very little attention available for staying awake. In effect, with the loss of attention (and interest) he slowly goes unconscious.

3. Before the end of the chapter, he is fast asleep.

Mario J. Giordano

Does this sound familiar? I'm sure this has happened to you. I know it has happened to me, many times. I used to think that reading in bed was the best tranquilizer or sleeping pill on the market. I never knew what was putting me to sleep until I understood the Golden Rule of Learning.

You can prove this out for yourself, too; either by observing your own behavior the next time you study or by recalling the many bad study sessions you've had in the past. You'll find - as I did - that the basic action that leads to failure-to-learn is the skipped-over word that was not understood.

HOW TO APPLY THE FIRST GOLDEN RULE OF LEARNING

Now you know the basic secret to learning - something relatively few people know. Now, here's how to use this information.

The *very first thing* to do is promise yourself, *from this day onward*, that you will never again pass a word you do not understand without first stopping to look up its meaning. Make it a compulsion. Refuse to accept words for which you do not have an immediate understanding. And the word "immediate" is important.

Secondly, buy several good dictionaries and place them in various rooms in your home. If you're a student, carry one with you to every class you attend. Always have a dictionary at your elbow.

Also, make it a point to buy (or develop) a glossary of technical terms for any subject you study. For instance, if you want to make your career in the business world, it is essential that you have a *general* glossary of business terms. Additionally, you should have a dictionary of *specific* terms in the specialized field of business in which you are interested.

If you intend to earn your living in real estate, get a good dictionary of real-estate terms. If you intend to become an accountant, get a good dictionary of accounting terms. Whatever field you are in as a career, or merely as a hobby, you should acquire - *as your basic tool for learning* - a good dictionary of technical terms for that field of study.

Not 'til then are you armed for fast learning and full understanding. Now, you merely *have to use* your dictionaries and glossaries to reach full understanding.

Thirdly, obey the first Golden Rule - **NEVER** (and I emphasize the word **NEVER**) *go past a word you do not fully understand.*

But, that's not the whole message. *HOW* we define words is equally important. It is the basis for our second Golden Rule of Learning:

DON'T DEFINE WORDS BY USING SYNONYMS

Many of us have gotten into the bad habit of defining a word by the use of synonyms. When we look up a word and we don't really understand what we read, we try to attach it to a synonym. Thereafter, we use the synonym instead of the word we looked up. The first word still remains misunderstood. Dullness and boredom still remain. What we failed to do is follow through and look up the "not-known" words *in the definition*. When I personally realized this, I hit upon my "closing-the-loop" described in FLM #7.

Remember, you cannot build a body of knowledge on a word you do not understand, and synonyms *aren't* the way. Get the word itself understood. Get the word itself used. Don't use synonyms in its place. Here is an example of what might happen when you do:

Say you came across the word "stellar" and after looking it up you used "*pertaining to stars*" as its meaning. Now, just imagine how many sentences using this word would throw you into confusion if you tried to use the synonym "star" in place of the word "stellar"!

Would you be accurate to say that an author's stellar writing was the author's writing pertaining to stars?

Remember, get the *word itself* defined. Own the word *itself*. Don't use synonym crutches to prop up your fuzzy thinking. Use the word itself in sentences. See how it applies to your life. This is how you get to "*own*" a word. This is how you become a clear, sharp, accurate thinker, which leads to the third Golden Rule of Learning ...

FULL UNDERSTANDING COMES FROM USING

A full understanding does not come from storing facts and definitions. It comes from using what you have learned. A full understanding, then, follows. You must use the word before you can *fully* understand it. Put action into all of your learning. Then you will realize what words *really* mean.

Use them in sentences. Use them in conversation. Insist on being as accurate as you can in using the words right. That's all there is to it.

Now, let's repeat the Golden Rules:

Rule #1: NEVER SKIP OVER A WORD YOU DO NOT FULLY UNDERSTAND. IF, DURING STUDY, YOU FIND YOURSELF CONFUSED OR UNABLE TO GRASP THE DATA, GO BACK TO THE POINT IN YOUR STUDY WHERE YOU WERE LAST UNCONFUSED. (Just before that point is a word you did not understand. Look up that word.)

Rule #2: NEVER PUT ANOTHER WORD IN THE PLACE OF THE WORD NOT UNDERSTOOD. THE ORIGINAL WORD REMAINS MISUNDERSTOOD.

Rule #3: FULL UNDERSTANDING COMES FROM USING THE DEFINED WORD.

Spend a few minutes mastering these rules. Make it a point to use them during your study of this report. Make sure there is no word in this report you cannot fully define.

Mario J. Giordano

Get yourself a dictionary *right now*. Place it beside yourself as you read on. Look up any word you find you cannot immediately understand or define. Not later - right then and there.

Be ruthless with yourself. Don't allow fuzzy thinking. Check, while you are studying these pages, that you remain ever alert and awake; that your concentration never wavers; that you have a full grasp of what you're learning.

Of course, how you use this FLM to make money or reach any other goal should be obvious to you by now.

ANY BODY OF KNOWLEDGE, FULLY MASTERED, CAN BE TURNED INTO MONEY.

Do you want to make money on the stock market? Then you must fully understand that body of knowledge. So, study it from a good book and from people who are successful at it.

But, during your study of the stock market, make sure you understand the meaning of every *one of its technical terms*. Through that understanding your chances of making money on the stock market become almost assured *if* you use what you learn.

Do you want to make money in real estate? Again, remember: you are still dealing with a body of knowledge. Learn about real estate by using this FLM. You *will* make more money in that field. Learn the words in accounting, and you can make money as an accountant. Learn the nomenclature about speculation in commodities, and you can make money as a speculator. The key word is "learn." And the basic law and rule of learning is "NEVER SKIP OVER A WORD YOU DO NOT FULLY UNDERSTAND."

FAST LEARNING METHOD #2

A FAST STUDY METHOD THAT GUARANTEES HIGH TEST SCORES

THIS SIMPLE METHOD MAKES YOU A FAST LEARNER BY SHOWING YOU HOW TO MAKE IT UNLIKELY FOR ANYONE (EVEN A TEACHER) TO ASK YOU A QUESTION YOU CANNOT ANSWER ON A TOPIC YOU'VE JUST STUDIED.

It sounds impossible; but, believe me, this Fast Learning Method (FLM) does just that. It guarantees high test scores. To better understand how, let's first look at what it takes to get a high score on tests – in reverse order. This is the same thing we looked at in FLM Number One, when we examined why people fail to learn. We now look at it positively instead of negatively.

Starting with the fifth step, know what probable questions might be asked in a test. Fourth, know the correct answers to these questions. Third, know all the facts in the study assignments (text) from which these test questions are made. Second, know a method for extracting these facts from the written material. And, first, know how written materials are formed from outlines of facts.

If you could know all these things, you'd never again have to fear any test. This FLM is designed to give you this knowledge. Before we get into the details, however, let me tell you where I first learned about this system.

HISTORY OF THE SYSTEM

After World War II, I was one of many veterans who took advantage of the *G.I. Bill of Rights*. I went back to school. The first two years of my undergraduate days were a disaster. I just couldn't get the hang of *how* to study or *what* to study. How to dig out important facts in my studies was a complete mystery to me. So, I never knew enough to make high marks on tests. My best efforts most often ended with a "C" grade or less.

I wasn't the only one having problems, either. Every veteran that started the freshman year with me was gone by the end of the sophomore year. I must admit, I almost dropped out myself – several times.

But, I was more fortunate than the others. There was a certain Economics Professor (one of the few great teachers I have known) who took an interest in me and became concerned about my failure to get the grades he thought I should.

He took me aside one day and told me that the only reason I wasn't making good grades was because *I never learned how good grades are made*. Then, he asked, "Where do you think my test questions come from?" I "hm'ed" and "uh'ed" my way to several feeble answers. But, he kept asking the question until I finally said, "From the important facts in the course." "From where do I get the facts of the course?" he continued. After a few wrong answers, I finally said the right one: "From your lectures and the chapters in the text."

Then, he told me that most teachers do the same. If I wanted to get good grades, I had to use this information to form study and learning routines. "Your study routines should parallel the professor's test-preparation routines." This is what he recommended:

1. Write down on a piece of paper *all the facts* from the chapter you are studying.

2. Make a question from each fact. Write these beside the respective fact.

3. Use these to study for the test.

He guaranteed that I would see an immediate improvement if I followed this system.

Now, even as I write this, it seems such a simple system for study that it couldn't possibly work. I thought the same thing at the time. I confess that I didn't put it to immediate use, and I continued receiving mediocre grades. When I finally got desperate, I decided to try it out. After all, what was there left to lose?

To make a long story short, this study system made it possible for me to finish my undergraduate days on the Dean's list – all B's and A's. I continued getting these grades throughout graduate school.

Now, let me say that, up to the time I began using this system - which I will shortly give to you in much greater detail - *I was just an average person making less than average grades*. This FLM *alone* was responsible for my finishing college. As a matter of fact, it has held me in good stead for many years since. Now, I'll pass it on to you. Use it. *It works!!*

THE SYSTEM FOR GUARANTEEING HIGH TEST SCORES

Since this FLM calls for you to study from study sheets that you make yourself, your first action will be to learn its format. Draw a pencil line down the middle of several sheets of lined paper. Put a heading on your first study sheet with an appropriate title. (Use the Chapter title.) Head the left column "Questions" and the right column "Answers."

Chapter One: ACCOUNTING PRINCIPLES

Questions	Answers
	The accounting equation is $A = L + P$
	Assets are things owned
	Etc.

Mario J. Giordano

Now, you are ready to start pulling facts from the chapter.

The chapter title is the first thing you start with. Write this at the top of your study sheet. Then, begin reading the first paragraphs. When you come to the first statement of fact, stop reading and write the fact on the answer side of your study sheet. Record *every fact* you come across in the same way until you reach the end of the section or chapter. That's the hardest part of your job. (NOTE: A complete review of FLM #6: "Flash Reading for Understanding" will give you the main parts of an author's outline and what you should look for under each part.) It's really very easy. You'll do it correctly the first time you try.

Now, you have finished your reading, extracted all the facts, and recorded them on your study sheet. This action, believe it or not, gives you the *answers to any questions that could he asked about the material in the chapter*. You are now ready for your next step.

Make a question out of each fact, and write that question on the left side of the study sheet, alongside its answer. For instance:

Chapter One: ACCOUNTING PRINCIPLES

Questions	Answers
What is the accounting equation?	The accounting equation is $A = L + P$
What are assets?	Assets are things owned
	Etc.

After you have transferred every fact to the right side of the study sheet and thought of an appropriate question for each fact on the left side, you have completed your study sheet for that chapter. You will never again have to read that chapter for the information that's in it.

Now, take your study guide to your next class. During the lecture, add to it any new data that the teacher may give. You will probably find you already knew the entire contents of his lecture and have more data on your study sheet than given in the entire lecture. That's the way it generally worked out for me.

When the teacher gives a new assignment, you repeat the same actions. You continue these actions for each assignment until test day. Now, here's how to study for tests.

On the day before the test, take out your study guide for each chapter. Put a piece of paper over the answers and *pre-test yourself*. Read a question. Answer it and then check your answer *immediately* against the right side of your study guide. Do this with each question until you come to the end of the guide.

How to Study and Master Any Subject – Quickly!

Additionally, while you move from question to question, put a check mark beside each one that gave you trouble. When you finish your first "go through" go back and review the troublesome questions. Get them right. Then, go through the entire list again. Continue this procedure until you are sure you *know* the answer to each question on the guide without peeking at the answer.

Just repeat this same routine for each chapter covered in the test. That's all there is to it. And I know of no better way to study for a test.

Here's another suggestion that could save you a lot of time studying for tests. Rather than do all your studying the night before the test, study each chapter thoroughly after the last lecture on that chapter. You'll not only be better prepared for the next chapter assignment; you'll also reduce your studying time the night before tests. It shouldn't take you more than 20 or 30 minutes to refresh your memory on fuzzy areas you might need help on.

On test day, you will walk into class certain that there is nothing the instructor could ask you that you don't already know. You may have a few doubts the first time you put this system to the test, but after you see how effective this FLM is, you will never again fear tests.

Let's repeat the steps in this system:

1) As you read, record all the facts you find on the "Answer" side of your study guide.

2) Make a question from each fact and write it on the "Question" side.

3) Update your study sheet during the class lecture.

4) Study by pre-testing yourself from your study guides. (For maximum learning, immediately reveal the answer after mentally answering each question. Check the ones that give you trouble.)

5) Review troublesome questions until you no longer need to check your answers.

6) Review entire list until fully learned.

7) Study only from study guides for tests.

That's all you have to do. But, don't let its simplicity fool you. It's one of the most effective learning methods you'll ever come across. Although at first it may not seem to speed up your learning, it will eventually prove to be one of the fastest learning methods of the eight I've compiled. After all, the shortest distance between two points is a straight line. In most cases, it's also the fastest. This FLM goes from Point #1 (I don't know the data) to Point #2 (I got an "A" on the test) in the most direct way I know. Try it out for yourself. You'll see.

Mario J. Giordano

FURTHER USE FOR THIS EASY STUDY SYSTEM

After you leave school - or if you have already left – and before you leave this planet, there will be many more bodies of knowledge you will have to master to survive. It's been estimated that the average person will return to school seven times in his lifetime before he leaves the labor force. This FLM will come in handy on each of these occasions. You won't ever have to give the excuse, "I'm pretty rusty; that's why I made a low grade."

Of course, there will be many other test-taking occasions outside of school that you'll have to go through. Civil service, college entrance, graduate preparation tests, test for licenses, job aptitude tests - are just a few. Use this FLM to prepare yourself for each one of these or, for that fact, *any body of knowledge you want to thoroughly learn.*

Fast Learning Method #3

Speed Learning Through Individualized Instruction

This simple method makes you a fast learner by showing you how to learn on your own - without classes and teachers - through this fool-proof method that hardly anyone knows about.

The biggest mistake you can make after leaving school is to think your formal schooling is finished and you now have all the data you'll need to succeed in life. This is far from the truth. Most of the data that you get in school - at least vocational data - will probably become obsolete within five years after you learn it. Technology is moving so fast today that, unless you keep up with the changes made, you'll soon find yourself on the labor trash heap.

This is the problem facing most job-holders today. How is it solved? Do you go back to school every other year to catch up on what you should know? This would be time consuming and costly - but mostly, *unnecessary*.

There is a solution in the form of an educational technology based on self-learning called individualized or "programmed" instruction. I call it I.I. for short. It comes in many forms, but the most useful to the average person is in book form.

Individualized instruction is based on scientifically sound findings of behavioral psychologists in their research on how people learn. About 15 years ago, these behavioral psychologists, because of what they found, came up with four major principles of effective learning. I.I. is based on these principles:

- The subject material should be presented in *small* doses and in *logical* order for learning to be effective.

- The learner must make an *active* response to each stimulus.

- The learner must know immediately if his response was correct.

- Each learner should work at his own speed.

Today, there are thousands of available I.I. books based on these four major principles of effective learning. They can be bought by anyone on practically any subject. And, believe me, some of the better ones can teach you as well, or better, than the average teacher in a classroom. This is because I.I. books - and there are good ones and bad ones - are based on the four major principles of effective learning. Few teachers bother to make sure that each of their lessons has the same basis. So, I.I. is worth looking into. Let's do it in a little more detail:

WHAT IS A PROGRAMMED TEXT?

First, the individualized instruction text (sometimes called a programmed text) is unlike any book you have ever read. It is mainly a conversation between a teacher (the author) and you. It is designed around a format of statements, questions, and answers. The most important parts are the questions. Your responses require an action by either writing answers on a separate piece of paper or performing some act that exposes the correct answer to you. After you have given your answer, there is some device - and there are several ways that this can be done - which immediately reveals to you whether your answer is correct. In other words, the results of your answer are *immediately* fed back to you.

Now, how are the programmed-instruction books superior to most of the classroom teaching you've had?

First of all, there is the strict standard against which programmed-instruction is tested before it is sold to the public. In most cases, a programmed text is not released unless it has been field-tested. In field-testing, the text must have a track record whereby 90% of the students receive 90% on their first try. In education, this is called the 90/90 criterion. It makes sure that the learning produced by the text has been tested over and over again until it is reasonably certain that people trying it for the first time can count on *mastering* it without too much trouble.

When you first discover I.I., you'll probably feel - as I did - that it's a second-hand way of learning, that it can't compete with professional teaching in the classroom. Let me debunk this right now. These books are written by professionally-trained course designers and teachers who know what the *science of learning* and the *art of teaching* are all about.

Your reaction to this might be, "Aren't the teachers in public education trained teachers, too?" I'm sorry to say that, on the college level, they're probably not. I'm currently teaching in a college where a Master's degree in a specialty field is the only requirement to teach. Whether the professor has been trained to teach is of secondary importance. That is why we generally find a subject-matter expert in front of a classroom, one who more-than-likely does not know how to teach or never received formal training in the science of learning. That's probably why lectures are, mostly, the only teaching method used. And, research has shown that lectures are mostly ineffective and unfruitful.

Let's put this statement to a test to see if it's true. Have you ever had a teacher who guaranteed that 90% of the class would receive a grade of "90" or better at the end of the course? Were you ever in a class where 90% of the students received an "A" as a final grade? More than likely, the answer to both questions is "NO," with rare exceptions here and there. However, in I.I., this guarantee is insisted upon. Any good programmed text has been field-tested to 90/90 before it is released. How many classroom teachers can say that?

But, does I.I. work? I can unconditionally state that it has worked for me and for many of my students. For instance, I've taught myself computer programming, writing, computer math, poetry, grammar, electronics, management, investments, and algebra - all on my own, through a programmed book, at my own rate of speed, and without the bother of attending classes at scheduled times or being exposed to inferior teaching.

Hundreds of my students can give you similar experiences. I recommend, as a matter of routine, to any student having trouble in any course to complete a programmed text in that course. I recommend other things, too, but they're covered in my other FLMs.

HISTORY OF INDIVIDUALIZED INSTRUCTION

As I mentioned before, individualized (programmed) instruction is based upon the laws of learning uncovered by behavioral psychologists, the most famous of which is Dr. B. F. Skinner of Harvard University. He developed the first *workable* teaching machine used in the early years of programmed instruction. Later, however, machines were dropped in favor of programmed books. One of Dr. Skinner's contributions is a behavioral law that states that a person tends to repeat an act that produces a pleasant result. Now, this statement is true, but *what* produces a pleasant result consistently, to all? Dr. Skinner never explained this to my full satisfaction. This law remained, for me, unused until I studied the works of L. Ron Hubbard (the founder of Scientology). A learning law that he formulated seems to parallel Dr. Skinner's but makes much more sense to the layman. Hubbard said that one tends to repeat pro-survival acts and avoid contra-survival acts. He goes on to say that one of the most basic *pro-survival* experiences is being *right* (correct) in our actions - the most basic *contra-survival* experience is being *wrong*.

With Hubbard's Law, you can now understand the importance of the 90/90 criterion. It insists that programmed courses be designed to give students only "wins" through *right* answers. These are pro-survival experiences.

Hubbard's "law" also agrees with Skinner's statement about pleasant results. Pleasure as defined by Hubbard is the emotion received from pro-survival acts. So, it all ties in nicely. One tends to learn better through - and feels pleasure from - a course that guarantees "wins." The reverse is also true. Now you can understand why so many people find schools unpleasant.

Another major learning law from behavioral psychologists states that knowing the *results* of one's actions must immediately follow the action if maximum learning is to take place. This means that the more you delay the feedback to the learner, the more confusing and uncertain learning becomes.

In I.I. textbooks, feedback about your answer immediately follows the act of answering. Not so in the average classroom. Teachers seldom, if ever, return test papers immediately. A delay of several days to a week is usually the custom. Skinner says that this is ineffective feedback with little or *no enforcing of learning*. Individualized instruction tries not to make this mistake.

LEARNING STRATEGIES IN INDIVIDUALIZED INSTRUCTION

There are two learning strategies generally used: forward chaining and backward chaining. The first teaches you the very basics of a skill and then, small step by small step, like links in a chain, moves you to the point where you master the entire skill. This is much like the method used to teach typing. First, the "home row" is taught. Other keys are then taught, followed by word-responses and so forth. Before long, a person can type without looking at the keys.

Another example of forward chaining would be the way children are taught to read and write. First they are taught the letters of the alphabet, which lead to words, then sentences, and so on.

Backward chaining is relatively new as a method of teaching. The best example I can give you of backward chaining is a programmed book written by Bobby Fisher, the Chess Champion, and programmed by S. Margulies and D. Mosenfielder. The book starts with the end of the match, showing you a chess situation where you have the other player checkmated. You're asked whether or not you have won. You answer "yes" or "no" and then turn the page to see if you're right. If you are wrong, you're told why. You're then told to repeat the step. If you answer correctly, you're given other situations involving the last move. This action is repeated until you fully know what "*check*" and "*mate*" mean.

Next, you're taught situations in which you are *two steps away* from checkmating your opponent, using the same format as before. When you complete this section of the program, you are moved into situations in which you are *three steps* away from checkmating. In the end, you are thinking in terms of four or five moves before checkmating. By this method of backward chaining, you become a pretty good chess player.

Whether the text uses backward chaining or forward chaining, the secret of its success is that each step (frame) is so small that you - going through the course - never have the feeling that you missed something. You hardly realize you are learning as much as you are.

Yes, I.I. is a highly effective learning system. There are several behavioral psychologists who, because of its success, have concluded that almost anything can be learned if the steps are small enough. Hubbard said the same thing when he stated, "The most difficult subject can be learned by anyone if the learning is done on small enough gradients." Add these two statements to this one making the rounds among educators: "About 95% of the populace can *MASTER ANY BODY OF KNOWLEDGE* if given enough *TIME*." The individualized instruction system will not only teach you in very small gradients, but provides you with all the time you need to master its contents. Wouldn't you say that's worth looking into?

WHERE TO FIND "PROGRAMMED" BOOKS

About this time, you should be very eager to go through an I.I. course, if you can find where to get one. The odd thing about I.I. is that, as soon as you become aware of its existence, you become amazed at *how many* programmed texts are available to the public.

Mario J. Giordano

Start your search at your local library. It probably stocks many books using the programmed format. Just ask your librarian about the programmed text on the course that you want. Be sure to say, "programmed text." I'm sure you won't be disappointed.

The best source I know, however, for seeing what is available in individually-paced instruction is a catalog written by Dr. Carl Hendershot. Your library probably has this catalog, also. It contains the most up-to-date listing of all available programmed texts on the market, in practically any subject. Hendershot tells you where to buy and what it will cost.

In the field of business alone, there are courses in accounting, banking, secretarial skills, hotel and restaurant training, insurance, management, sales, retailing, computers, and others.

In the subject of English, practically any text dealing with any part of English, from capitalization to writing prose, can be bought.

Foreign languages, too, are thoroughly covered with courses in French, German, Greek, Hebrew, Italian, and many others.

Mathematics, as a field, has many "programmed" courses from basic arithmetic to sophisticated courses in logarithms, trigonometry, calculus, and on up.

The sciences are also represented with courses in Biology, Chemistry, Physics, and so forth.

I doubt if there is a general-education subject for which a programmed-instruction text is not available on the open market. Dr. Hendershot's catalog practically lists them all.

(Editor's Note: As was previously stated in the Forward to this book, Prof. Giordano is speaking to us from 1975. The internet didn't exist then and the only way to find these materials was to either go to bookstores or to libraries. Today, there are many sources on-line for Individualized or Programmed Instruction, as well as on-line courses in practically every subject imaginable. A simple search will provide you with thousands of sources to improve your knowledge at little to no cost.)

WHY USE I.I.?

As I said previously, the major reason for using individualized instruction is because it's such a darn good way to learn – far superior in many ways to attending classes. But, there are other reasons.

First, there is the cost factor. Many courses listed in Hendershot's catalog are less than $10, with some of the most expensive ones not more than $50. Where else could you be sure of mastering a subject at such low prices?

Another reason for using I.I. concerns the time factor. With I.I., there is no such thing as having to study at certain times of the day, during certain days of the week, for certain months of the year. With I.I., you move at your own rate of speed. You can take a break anytime and for as long as you want. How could you ever duplicate that in a classroom?

Finally, one of the minor reasons for using this system – one most often heard from students who have used it - has to do with competition. Some people don't like the competitive atmosphere of the classroom. They don't like being compared with other students to determine what grade they will receive. (Believe it or not, this is a major method used by teachers today for determining the grade of a student. It has to do with the bell-shaped curve. I don't agree with it. There should be only one way to determine whether you have learned a subject: can you demonstrate that you have mastered the data? Can you apply what you have learned? This is what I.I. grades you on.

HOW CAN I.I. MAKE YOU A FAST LEARNER?

This should now be quite obvious to you. Since you can move at your own rate of speed, there is nothing holding you back to absorbing the most knowledge in the least amount of time possible *for you*.

I completed an entire grammar course - one that takes an entire year in high school - in less than three days of intensive work. And believe me, I *learned* grammar.

Whenever you want to find out about a body of knowledge, your first action is to get a programmed text in that subject and spend a couple of intensive hours with it. This is usually enough to give you the amount of data you need to make good decisions involving that body of knowledge.

Try it. See how quickly you can impress your friends with your knowledge in many subjects. All it takes is a few hours of your time on each. You may even find to your surprise that you can now learn enough data in a subject - on your own - to be classified as an expert.

With programmed courses, you can *thoroughly learn* many bodies of knowledge without ever once attending a class. Just think of what this means to you in keeping up with your field. You will never again have to fear becoming obsolete. In one short weekend, you can master the contents of the latest data in your field. That's an FLM worth knowing!

FAST LEARNING METHOD #4

UNDERSTANDING BY DEMONSTRATING WITH OBJECTS

THIS SIMPLE METHOD MAKES YOU A FAST LEARNER BY SHOWING YOU HOW TO PUT POWER IN YOUR STUDY EFFORTS THROUGH THE SIMPLE USE OF BRIC-A-BRAC FOUND IN ANY HOME.

Most of us have problems with words - both written and spoken - because they are symbols of things, not the things themselves. So, before you can learn by the use of symbols, you must know what the object of the symbol looks like, feels like, and so on. Also, you must know what symbol represents each part of the object.

For instance, if you never saw an automobile, and I told you to put the gear shift in "drive," how much understanding would you have? Practically none.

If you came upon an object you never saw before - let's say that you just landed on this planet and you've come upon your first sight of a tree - you wouldn't need a symbol to represent what you are looking at to learn about it. You'd go up to the tree, feel it, climb it, or you might even taste a leaf from it. In that way, you would learn first-hand what a tree tastes like, feels like, and looks like. Problems pop up only when you have to communicate these experiences to someone else, without the object at hand. You have to communicate the sight, the feel, and the taste "symbolically."

Communicating with symbols instead of the object itself will definitely cause you confusion and misunderstanding if you do not have exactly the same meanings for the symbols used as the person you're talking to.

And, that's the trouble with much of our education. It mainly teaches about things in the absence of the things themselves. In many cases, we are taught to do something without being asked to demonstrate that we know how to do it. Learning, then, becomes top-heavy in *significances* (meanings) and lacks the better form of learning - looking, touching, using, etc.

To best understand a subject, you should learn with the objects and by the actions the subject is about. Teaching a person about a particular object - such as motor repair when he doesn't have a motor to work on - never really gets the subject across. The simple solution would be to supply the object and teach the actions that are to be studied. This is not always possible, though.

For instance, it's difficult to bring a bridge into the classroom where you're teaching bridge erecting. It's also too expensive to bring a computer into a classroom when you're teaching computer technology.

The less we learn with objects, the more we have to use symbols. Whenever we're forced to do this, we make understanding that much more difficult.

So, some ways are better than others to learn by. These ways can be put on a scale ranging from best to worst. There *is* an actual "scale-of-learning" that progressively moves from the most difficult way to learn up to the fastest way. At the top of the scale is learning about an object first-hand, without the use of symbols. At the bottom of the scale is learning about an object entirely through the use of symbols. The scale looks something like this:

1. Using the object to know about it. (matter)

2. Sensing the actual object. (looking, hearing, touching)

3. Thinking about the object. (mental pictures)

4. Using symbols in place of the object. (words, numbers, etc.)

In other words, the actual tree is more real to you (using the senses) than a mental image picture of a tree (thinking about trees). Also, a mental image picture - going down the scale - is more real to you than the symbol, "tree." Here, the symbol has to be translated mentally into a mental image picture before understanding is complete.

The further we go up the scale in designing a method of learning, the more effective the learning method becomes. If you only learned about fixing automobiles by reading about them, without ever seeing or touching an automobile engine, you'd wind up with a lot of theory, meanings, and significances. You would not have learned how to handle the object itself. So, to best teach yourself anything, you must add the mass of the object to the significances and meanings of the theory. In this way, learning becomes far more complete than dealing with only the symbols in a body of knowledge.

If you understand the learning scale, you'll understand the full meaning of: "One picture is worth a thousand words." But, more than that, you'll know why the object itself is worth a thousand pictures.

Now, I've taken a long time to get to the point. I did this purposely because I didn't know for sure if you know the reasons and theory for what follows. What I've just said is the basis for this Fast Learning Method (FLM). Let's finally get on with it.

ADDING MATTER TO LEARNING

As I said before, it is difficult to bring a building into a classroom to teach architects about construction. Likewise, it's difficult to provide bridges, farms, stars, and the like. Something has to take their place in the learning of bodies of technology about these items.

Unfortunately, some educators think that words and their meanings are all that is necessary to take the place of the objects they symbolize. If this were so, misunderstanding of lectures and concepts would be unheard of. There wouldn't be a need for dictionaries to tell you what the symbols mean. The subject of English - the

Mario J. Giordano

one most studied during your school years - would not be the failure it is. We wouldn't have high school graduates who could barely read the newspaper. Math wouldn't be the mystery it is.

Now, you can appreciate why the three Golden Rules of Learning, as described in FLM #1, are so important. They are the very basics to learning in a symbol-based educational system.

So, how do we make learning *easier* in a symbol-based system when it is impractical and sometimes impossible to have the objects available while learning is going on? It's really very simple. It's so simple that it's hard to believe that it works.

USE A SUBSTITUTE OBJECT!

Oddly enough, using and handling a *substitute* object while learning with *symbols increases understanding and speeds up learning*. And, it doesn't matter *what* object you use to take the place of the real thing. It can be a thimble, a match stick, a paper clip, a button, a piece of chalk, or any other small item that you can find.

To put it another way, if you are learning how to drive an automobile and you don't have an automobile available, use a button to represent a steering wheel, a paper clip to represent a gear shift, a piece of chalk to represent a brake, a hairpin to represent a clutch, and so forth. Don't laugh as I did when I first heard this. Try it. It works!!

When you come across written symbols representing objects, you'll learn much faster if you *perform the action* called for *directly on the substitute objects*. For instance, if the words say, "Push in the clutch and place the gear shift in low, "press a finger on the hair pin (clutch) and move the paper clip (gear shift) to the "first position." Do you see what you're doing? You're adding actions to your learning. *You're going through the motions*. You're also putting mass back into learning.

The important thing to remember is to handle the substitute object in much the same way you would the actual object itself. You are, in effect, learning by doing. And it works!

So, when you're studying, have a small box of bric-a-brac handy. Dump the items on the desk in front of you. As you read, pick up a piece of bric-a-brac and have it represent the object you're reading about. Do the same for other words. Finger these objects as you study the body of knowledge. Demonstrate what you're studying through the use of the *substitute* objects - it will amaze you how fast you learn the concepts you are studying.

You'll understand much better why Napoleon was defeated if you were to lay out the Waterloo Battlefield with items from your box of bric-a-brac. It's much easier to follow the step-by-step actions when you manipulate actual objects than it is to mentally manipulate written symbols.

So, try it. You'll see that it's not as silly as it first sounds. And, it's logical, too. Remember the learning scale? The closer you get (in your studies) to the objects and the actions that the subject is about, the better the learning system and the more you'll be able to understand that subject. Why handicap yourself with just symbols? Substitute objects for those words. It's not as good as using the real objects - but substitute mass is far better than substitute symbols.

Fast Learning Method #5

Fast Learning by Removing Unimportant Data

This simple method makes you a fast learner by showing you how to quickly absorb the basics of any subject and give yourself a bedrock foundation of what you want to know.

Closely related to the problem of too much use of symbols in learning is the problem of "too many facts" in the subject - all seemingly of equal importance. This happens whenever you study a body of knowledge through a teacher - or an author - that presents the material in such a way that everything seems of equal importance. You are probably being instructed by a person *who has never used that subject in the actual world of work*. An accounting teacher who has never been an accountant makes accounting very difficult to learn.

It's a strange thing. Whenever you have a person teaching vocational subjects who got his knowledge from schools or books only, you have a teacher who will make every fact in that body of knowledge of equal importance. The paint on the car is as important as the clutch, which is as important as the floor mat, which is as important as the motor, and so on.

Is it any wonder that students become confused about studying for a test in a subject where everything is of equal importance to everything else? That happens often in too many classrooms. We have business, teaching future secretaries, who have never worked in an office themselves. We have teachers, teaching accounting to future accountants, who have never been accountants themselves. And so it goes.

What do you do about a subject that confuses and overwhelms you with facts and data? Well, the one thing you do, if you are ever to understand and use that subject, is to select out all the unimportant data from the body of knowledge so that only the important items remain.

For instance, if I were to help a student who was unfortunate enough to have been taught how to drive a car from one who never drove before – who loaded the student down with insignificances – I would ask the student, "What don't you have to know to drive that car?" After I got an answer, I would ask the question again. I would continue asking this *same question* after each answer until there were no more answers. What is left are the important data you need to know to drive the car. All unimportances have been selected out.

In my use of this technique, I have found that most people act the same at first. Their data is so unaligned and so overwhelming that they can't grab hold of one significant fact. Eventually, they give an answer. It's easier after that.

The student might first answer, "The paint on the fender." But, after a while, they are answering, "the motor," the "differential" and so forth. I follow each answer with the same question, insisting on answers until we get down to only the essential data that needs to be known to drive a car.

This system really rehabilitates a person's understanding of a body of knowledge, and you can use it on yourself just as effectively. Whenever a body of knowledge seems confusing or overwhelming to you, ask yourself the question, *"What don't I have to know to perform the actions of this subject?"* Continue asking this same question and answering honestly, over and over again, until you reduce the body of knowledge to its bare essentials. It will startle you how clear the data becomes. All the items align themselves properly, reducing the body of knowledge to its bare essentials. That's all you want to know and that's what this FLM is all about.

Now, don't think that this little Fast Learning Method will not come in handy. There are a great many teachers who are teaching and authors who are writing textbooks who have never performed in the subject they are teaching or writing about - more than I would care to mention. It is impossible for you to go through a school curriculum today without coming across them. So, learn to use this little FLM. It is a true, fast-learning method. It will come in handy more than once in your lifetime.

Mind you, this is not a way to pass tests. Use FLM #2 for that. This one will unconfuse and align data so that you can use the subject matter.

FAST LEARNING METHOD #6

FLASH READING FOR UNDERSTANDING

THIS SIMPLE METHOD MAKES YOU A FAST LEARNER BY SHOWING YOU HOW TO QUICKLY UNDERSTAND ANY WRITTEN DOCUMENT. YOU'LL QUICKLY AND EASILY ABSORB WHOLE BOOKS.

Reading is one of the three basic skills on which all other skills are based. The other two are, of course, writing and math. But reading is, by far, used more than the other two skills combined. So, if you want to advance in your career and life, you *must* become a good reader.

This Fast Learning Method (FLM) will help you greatly in all your reading, especially the kind you do every day with newspapers, magazines, novels, and non-fiction. This level of reading requires that you scan the written page quickly, but, at the same time, not miss its main ideas. Therefore, we are talking about a FLM designed to make you a master reader, not a master studier. Both skills do overlap, somewhat, though. As a master reader you'll need ...

1. The ability to ferret out only the main ideas of what you read;
2. To eliminate all the unnecessary words in what you read; and,
3. To boil down the main ideas into compact concepts.

As a master reader, you'll then be able to quickly extract the vital points from the written page, and condense them into concepts that you'll remember.

FLASH SCANNING A BOOK TO UNDERSTAND IT BEFORE YOU READ IT

This report is a typical written document, containing many main thoughts. But, before I wrote it, I sat down and outlined what I wanted to say. This outline contains all the main thoughts that I wanted to include. What you are really doing when you read it is searching for these ideas or main thoughts, whether you realize it or not.

The author's outline, therefore, is the key to flash reading any written document. You have to learn to look for - and extract - the author's outline. That's where you find the main ideas and facts - in the title, part headings, chapter headings, paragraph headings, topic sentences, and so forth.

If you were to make these headings into questions - and here's the trick to flash reading - and read for their answers, you would be reading with purpose. By turning the title of a book into a question, you'll know what you are looking for when you read the book. For instance, a title of a book, *Total Fitness*, would be formed into the question, "*How do I become totally fit?* " By the end of the book, you should have your answer.

Alternately, by making the chapter heading into a question, you purposely point to what you should know by the time you reach the end of the chapter. As an example, *Chapter Five - "Your Pulse and Your Fitness,"* would be changed to *"How does my pulse determine my fitness?"* By changing paragraph headings into questions in the same way, you'll find out what you should knew by the time you reach the end of the paragraph. And so it goes throughout the entire document.

The main trick to this method of fast reading, therefore, is to make questions out of the author's headings and to flash read for *answers only*.

Before you read a book, study a lesson, or look into any body of knowledge, your reading will be more purposeful and fruitful if you form the key questions *before* you start. Getting the questions answered extracts the main ideas of the document. Getting these main ideas out of the document is the *main purpose* for reading. When you come to the answer to a question, you stop reading. There is no need to wade through more unnecessary verbiage.

HOW EACH PART OF THE AUTHOR'S OUTLINE TELLS YOU WHAT TO LOOK FOR

As I said previously, an author first outlines his work before he writes. This outline eventually becomes chapter headings, paragraph headings, summaries, and so forth. These are the main thoughts. Let's take them, one at a time, and find out what to expect from each.

THE TITLE

Nowhere else can you better find the main theme of a book than in its title. It contains the entire theme of the book condensed into one line. This is the author's main message - that is, if he is not being too "cute" with his title.

Hemmingway's *For Whom The Bell Tolls* reveals his entire theme in that one line. When you finish reading his book, you should have learned the moral that every man's action will, in some way, affect the lives and actions of all other living things. Therefore, a person should be careful of his insistence that he be unfettered in his actions.

Re-write the title to read, *For Whom Does The Bell Toll?* By the end of the book, you'll have your answer - they toll for you.

TABLE OF CONTENTS

The table of contents is a list of main ideas in the order in which they are taken up - one thought leading to the understanding of the next. Study the table of contents to determine how the main theme is broken down into its parts. When you turn each into a main-idea question, you add purpose and direction to your reading.

THE INTRODUCTION

Mario J. Giordano

In the introduction, the author generally explains his purpose for writing what follows. This gives the reader valuable information about the main ideas of the document. Generally, the author will tell you what you are about to read, in a paraphrasal form. This, too, will give you direction in your reading.

FLASH READING THE CHAPTERS

Just like the book itself, the chapter, too, is pre-outlined before it is written. The trick is to use the chapter outline to extract its main ideas and thoughts.

Firstly, read the chapter title. Sitting there at the top of the page, it practically screams out to you what the chapter is about and sometimes much more. Re-word the chapter title so it is a question. Then, read 'til you find the answer. *That's your purpose.*

Many authors also write an introductory paragraph before getting on with the main thoughts in a chapter. A close inspection of the introductory paragraph will tell you exactly what to look for. But more than that, it probably tells you how it relates to the previous chapters in the text.

Secondly, next to the chapter title in importance are the section headings. They break down the chapter into main-thought parts. The answer to a question worded from a section heading is answered within that section. Look for that answer as you flesh read the section. Disregard all unnecessary words and sentences that do not fit your purpose.

Thirdly, the paragraph headings, found in many school texts, make great questions. They give you the main topic of the paragraphs, boiled down to a single phrase. Flash reading for the answer to these questions *really* speeds up your reading phenomenally!!

Fourthly, the most important sentences in the chapter are the topic sentences of each paragraph. A good writer uses one thought or idea for each paragraph. It is almost always in the first sentence of the paragraph. These are the topic sentences. A flash-read of these sentences will determine whether or not you have reached the answer to the question made from the paragraph headings. A quick jump from topic sentence to topic sentence can give you a fast grasp of a section and the answers you are looking for.

Lastly, many books contain a summary at the end of each chapter. Before you come to it, however, you should have already answered the questions made from the chapter title, section headings, paragraph headings, and so forth. The summary should be used as a check on whether you reached the correct answers to your flash-read questions. All the main thoughts of the chapter are located here. In effect, it is exactly what the author thought was important and what he wrote about.

So, you see, the key to flash reading with understanding is to first have an exact purpose and direction for your reading. You get this by turning all headings into questions and you read for answers only. Here's how in detail.

THE MECHANICS OF FLASH READING

Before you read in detail, first make questions from the title and the chapter headings and write these questions on a sheet of paper. Then, read the introduction to get a full understanding of how the book is put together. Look at the table of contents to see its structure. Then, turn to Chapter One.

Move on to the chapter introduction to get a feel of what's contained in the chapter. Make a question from the section or paragraph heading; then scan the material between this heading and the next. As soon as you come to the answer, write it on your paper and stop any further reading in that section.

Move on to the next heading. Make a question from it. Record the question on your paper. Flash read for its answer. Stop reading when you have your answer. Continue in this way through the chapter. Always remember, though, that the main thought of the chapter must also be answered as a check of your understanding.

If, at the end of the chapter, you can answer the question made from the chapter title you know that you have not only read the entire chapter as quickly as it can be studied, but you also have a full understanding of what the author wrote.

This is the fastest way I know to read for *maximum understanding*. It is fast because it is based on *directed* reading. There is no guessing about what will come from your reading, nor is there unnecessary reading of insignificant data. Directed reading speeds learning through the use of pre-recorded questions that must be answered by the end of the reading. So we read for answers only.

Read paragraphs to get the answer to paragraph questions;

Combine paragraph answers to get answers to chapter questions;

Combine chapter answers to get answers to section questions;

And, combine section answers to get answers to theme questions.

This is a complete system for reading that leaves nothing to chance and will leave you, the reader, with a thorough understanding of what you have read.

Fast Learning Method #7

MINI-COURSES FROM YOUR DICTIONARY

THIS SIMPLE METHOD MAKES YOU A FAST LEARNER BY SHOWING YOU HOW TO GET A QUICK MINI-COURSE OF ANY SUBJECT THROUGH AN ALMOST UNKNOWN USE OF THE DICTIONARY.

Most of what we have to learn in life has been placed in symbolic form (words), and most of these symbols (words) are contained in a good dictionary. It holds true, therefore, that the dictionary is an enormous source of information *comprising complete bodies of knowledge*. Moreover, these bodies of knowledge have been stripped of all unnecessary filler words and reduced to brief descriptions. Only the essential words needed to explain meanings have been included. Consequently, thousands of subjects - in mini-course format - are contained in the dictionary. But, they are scattered throughout the dictionary like pellets shot from a shotgun. How to un-scatter the data is answered by this Fast Learning Method (FLM).

Here, you will learn to extract complete bodies of knowledge from the dictionary, in compact form, that you can quickly study and absorb. I call this action, for want of a better name, "*closing the loop to understanding*." Here's how it works.

CLOSING THE LOOP TO UNDERSTANDING

Briefly, what you have to do is to define the word or words in the subject's title. Do it in ruthless detail through this step-by-step procedure:

1. Open the dictionary to the page containing the word you want defined.

2. Select the most appropriate definition from the ones given - the one that comes closest to your fuzzy understanding of the subject.

3. As you read the selected definition, mentally check to see if you *understand each word is used in the definition*. (Don't skip this one. It's very important.)

4. Now, select out and write down on a sheet of paper all the words from the definition for which you did not have an *immediate* understanding. (If you had to mentally search for the meaning, you didn't know the word well enough to use as a base for other information.)

5. Look up and define each word in the main definition that was not understood, and write the definition beside the word defined.

6. Repeat steps one to five for each word not understood until you close the loop to understanding the original definition.

In brief, you are defining a key word which leads to other key words in the subject you do not understand. You define all these words - in turn - using the same ruthless format – understanding each word in each definition. Sooner or later, the last word defined will lead you back to the main definition and miraculously close the loop to understanding. For instance:

Let's suppose that one day you ask your English teacher, "What is the purpose of my having to take a literature course?" He states to you, very briefly, "'to give you culture."

Later on in the day you realize that, although he gave you an answer, you didn't understand it. The word "culture" was not fully understood.

So, you look it up, and you find:

CULTURE: "Enlightenment and excellence of taste acquired by intellectual and aesthetic training."

Now, if you are like I am, you still will not know what culture means. The definition itself is not clear. It contains too many abstract terms. For instance:

What does "*enlightenment*" mean?

What does "*excellence*" mean?

What does "*taste*" mean in this definition? (It certainly has nothing to do with taste buds.)

What does "*intellectual*" mean?

What does "*aesthetic*" mean?

We still have a problem here. We don't know what the word "*culture*" means because there are several words within the definition that are vague in meaning. So, in keeping with the rules of this FLM, let's look up each "not-understood" word and get it thoroughly defined. You'll find this step easier to grasp if you use the outline form. This is how I closed the loop on "*culture*."

1. CULTURE: "Enlightenment and excellence of taste acquired by intellectual and aesthetic training."

A. DEFINITION OF ENLIGHTENMENT: "*Spiritual insight*; being given knowledge." (I, personally, had to look up the words *spiritual* and *insight* in order to understand enlightenment.)

    a. *Spiritual*: "Pertaining to an entity that gives life. (soul; the "I")"

    b. *Insight:* "Power to see into the essence of things."

Mario J. Giordano

So, I guess "enlightenment" means attaining knowledge through the life-giving entity (soul) which has the power to see into the essence of things.

B. DEFINITION OF EXCELLENCE: "Superiority; surpassing others."

To be cultured, then, makes us a cut above the average person.

C. DEFINITION OF TASTE: "Critical judgment or appreciation."

D. DEFINITION OF INTELLECTUAL: "The power of KNOWING distinguished from the power to feel. The capacity for rational or intelligent thought."

I had to look up the words "*intelligent*" and "*rational*" because I couldn't give an *immediate* definition.

Intelligent: "The capacity to apprehend facts, their propositions, and their relations and to reason about them." (Here I had to look up the word REASON.)

Reason: "Thinking in an orderly, *rational* way."

I was about to look up the word "rational," but here it appears in the definition of "reason." I know now that I am about to close the loop of understanding for the word "*intelligent*."

b. Rational: "Having understanding and reason."

Now, the definitions of the word "reason" and the word "rational" sort of closes the loop of understanding within themselves. "Reason" is thinking in an orderly, *rational* way; and "rational" means having *reason* and understanding.

So, we've now closed the loop for the term "intellectual," which we find means the development of the thinking part of us - rather than the feeling part of us - in a way that will allow us to look at data and reason correctly about them.

E. DEFINITION OF AESTHETIC: "The sensitivity to the beautiful."

This last word closes the loop of understanding for the word "culture". We have defined every fuzzy word within the definition. Now, we can define the word culture in our own words:

CULTURE: "Getting to understand knowledge (data) through the power to see the essence of things and developing critical judgement or appreciation that is superior to that of the average person. This comes about by being trained to develop the power to "know" through the development of rational thinking and reasoning. This is also done by being trained to recognize, and be sensitive to, the beautiful things in life."

Well, that's how it is done. Now, if you still do not know the meaning of the word "culture," it's because there are some words in its definition that you still do not understand. To get the full meaning, you will have to go through this whole exercise yourself, studying each word in each definition that you do not understand. Your understanding will come only *after each word associated with the word culture is thoroughly defined and understood.*

Let me give you another example from my own experience. I was sitting in a faculty meeting one day, listening to an English professor complain about the lack of understanding his students had about grammar. I have heard this complaint many times in my teaching years, but it suddenly dawned on me that I, too, didn't know what he meant by "grammar." I had to look up the word, which was a little embarrassing. This is what it took to close the loop of understanding for the word, "grammar."

GRAMMAR: "The study of the classes of words, their inflections, function, and relation in sentences."

Now, going through this definition, I eventually found out that "classes-of-words" meant nouns, pronouns, verbs, and so on. But, to thoroughly understand the word "grammar" I would have to understand the definition of *each* class of word.

But, let's go on. The next word I came across that gave me trouble was the word, "inflection." So, I had to look it up. This is what I found:

INFLECTION: "The change of form that words undergo to mark such distinctions as those of *CASE, GENDER, NUMBER, TENSE, PERSON, MOOD,* or *VOICE.*"

Believe it or not, I had to look up every word underlined in this definition before I understood the word, "inflection." So, you see how nitty-gritty this thing can get.

The word "sentence" in the original definition was never thoroughly understood either. So, I looked it up and found that it mainly deals with another vaguely understood word - syntax. By defining syntax (the way words are put together to form phrases, clauses, or sentences), I finally found out what a sentence is. And, in turn, I finally found out what "grammar" is all about.

In those three words - classes, inflections, and syntax - are contained all the symbols and definitions that were required by me before I could understand the technology of grammar.

I can't help feeling that if some of our English instructors would insist on each student closing the loop of understanding for the technology of grammar as I did - we would have fewer illiterates and many more people who could write intelligently.

To make my point more solid, let me give you one more example.

Mario J. Giordano

I was forced to look up the word "*logic*" one day after I asked a philosophy professor to define it for me. All I got was a confusion of words. The dictionary's definition was no better. Let me demonstrate why logic is so confusing and so difficult to learn by showing you what I found.

LOGIC: "A _science_ that deals with the _cannons_ and the _criteria_ of _validity_ of _inference_ and _demonstration_. _Normative_ principles of reasoning."

The underlined words are the ones I, personally, had to look up before I could even approach the understanding of the technology called *logic*. But worse than this, the philosophy professor's definition (a body of knowledge that he actually teaches) was *incorrect*! He didn't even know the definition of the subject he had studied and taught for years. How could he possibly teach it *rationally*?

I can give you case-after-case and example-after-example that would fully prove to you how unknown this little system-for-learning is. People not only do not go into the dictionary for the definitions of simple words, but they never even dream of the thousands of mini-courses contained therein.

So, this is the *secret of using a dictionary powerfully*. With this secret, you can, in a very short time, get a complete working knowledge of an entire subject. Here, too, is another piece of gold for you.

HOW TO USE THIS FLM

First, and without delay, close the loop of understanding for all your current activities.

If you have a job, then define the title of your job and all the words in that definition. The result will be a job description you can really work with.

If you're taking a course in school, define the course title and all the words within the title, and you will have a comprehensive understanding of the entire body of knowledge.

If you're pursuing a curriculum in school, define the curriculum title and all the words in the definition. You'll find out what you should be able to do upon graduation.

If you're looking around for a career that you might like, define the names of each career that strikes your fancy and the words within the definitions. When you're finished, you'll be able to select that career that best fits your talents.

And so it goes - whatever your current interests or hobbies are, define the words involved and you will be able to *perform the actions* much more quickly.

There will also be many occasions when you'll want to know much more clearly what the other fellow is saying. For instance, what are the interests of "that certain person" you would like to know better? Give yourself a mini-course in each of his/her interests. You will be surprised, thereafter, how easy it is to talk to that person.

What are the interests and training of your boss? A brief trip into the dictionary for a mini-course will give you all the data you'll need to get him interested in you.

If your boss likes golf and you don't know anything about it, give yourself a mini-course. It will give you enough data and understanding of the sport to talk intelligently about it. If he's human, like the rest of us, he'll *like* you better because you *like* something *he likes*. Get the point?

Though this FLM is little in scope, it is huge in results. There is no other way to more quickly understand an entire body of knowledge than "closing the loop to understanding."

FAST LEARNING METHOD #8

TRICKS TO MEMORIZING: IT'S EASY WHEN YOU KNOW HOW

THIS SIMPLE METHOD MAKES YOU A FAST LEARNER BY SHOWING YOU HOW TO USE A FEW SIMPLE TECHNIQUES FOR REMEMBERING WHOLE LISTS OF DATA YOU WILL AUTOMATICALLY RECALL EVEN MONTHS AFTER YOU'VE LEARNED THEM.

It's a known fact that the mind best remembers something new when it is associated with something already known and stored in the memory banks. Most of the memorizing systems that you come across are based on this fact. Three of the best are:

- Memorizing through association;
- Memorizing through mental picturing; and
- Memorizing through mnemonics.

The first two are more effective when they are combined in a single system. But, they do work individually and, I might add, most effectively.

The first usually teaches you how to memorize a list of ten or twenty items after only once hearing or seeing the list. When you demonstrate this extremely simple memorizing technique to your friends, expect to see startled faces. My students thought I was a mental giant until I showed them how *anyone* can learn it *in five minutes*. Here it is in detail:

MEMORIZING THROUGH ASSOCIATION

There will be many occasions when you'll need to memorize lists of items. Mostly, they have to be memorized in a certain order. Now, you can do this the hard way by reading the list over and over again until it becomes fixed in your mind. This may take hours, however. There is a much shorter way.

The first thing to do is *pre*-memorize a list of ten items that you can associate by *sound* with the *numbers* from one to ten. For instance, my pre-memorized list looks like this:

      For the number *one*, I picture a *woman*. (Notice the "W" sound for both the number *one* and the word *woman*.)

      For number *two*, I picture a *tulip*. Note again the sameness of sound.

For number *three*, I picture a *THREad*.

For *4, phone; 5, file; 6, sink; 7, leaven (flat dough); 8, ape; 9, knife and 10, tent*.

How to Study and Master Any Subject – Quickly!

Don't pre-memorize this list if it doesn't sound natural to you. Think up a list of your own. But it *is* necessary to pre-memorize a list because you need each item to form a mental-image picture that will connect with an item you are trying to memorize.

As an example, here's an arbitrary list of objects that I will demonstrate with to show you the mechanics of this system. Our objective, remember, is to memorize the entire list in the order given.

stick

book

typewriter

can

razor

skate

apple

pole

shoe

feather

To memorize the first item – stick –make a mental image picture of a woman (the object we pre-memorized to represent number one) holding a stick in her hand. This fixes the first item in your mind beside the number one. Just thoroughly picture the woman holding the stick. Thereafter, all you need do is think of "one." Mentally attached to it is the mental-image picture of a woman carrying a stick. That's all there is to it. That's how the mind indexes data, and that's the basis of this memorizing system.

It works backwards, too. Picture the stick and the woman holding it will emerge. This will tell you that it is the first item on the list.

To memorize the second item - book - make a mental image picture of a tulip lying across a book; when this becomes fixed in your mind - it takes just a few seconds - you have memorized the second item.

To memorize the third item - typewriter - make a mental image picture of a thread of yarn draped across the typewriter keys.

To memorize the fourth item, make a mental image picture of a phone balancing precariously on a can.

For item #5, picture a razor cutting through a wooden file cabinet.

For item #6, mentally place a skate in a sink.

For item #7, picture an apple in some unleavened dough.

For item #8, picture an ape climbing a pole.

For item #9, mentally stab the knife through a shoe.

And, for item #10, picture a feather at the entrance to a tent.

That's all there is to it. It's very easy to do, even the first time you try it.

Now, the best demonstration of the effectiveness of this system would be to tell you about what just happened as I was dictating this material to my secretary. I have demonstrated this system of memorizing to many people, but she never heard of it. To test me out, she asked me to name the items I just dictated backward. The result was, as usual, a startled person. Now, you can do the startling. You will be able to recite the list backward, forward, by number or by item.

Here it is again. First memorize a list of ten items that you will thereafter associate with the numbers from one to ten. Then, make a mental-image picture of these numbered items with any object that you want to remember. It's as simple as that.

Try it out right now. I'll bet that you memorize a list in less than five minutes. I will also bet that you will be able to name the objects by number, backwards, or even randomly.

MEMORIZING NAMES THROUGH ABSURD MENTAL PICTURES

I've always been bad with names; and to a teacher, that can be critical. People just don't like being called, "Hey, you!" In the past I tried to hide the fact that I forget names, but I was usually unsuccessful. So, I learned this simple method. I suggest you do the same. It will save you many embarrassing moments in your social life.

Whenever you want to remember a person's name, be immediately conscious of what the name reminds you of, or what it sounds like, or what the person looks like. In some way, associate this with the person himself.

For instance, I was once introduced to a very important man named Mr. Rosenwasser. How do you suppose I memorized his name? I associated it with two objects: a rose and a washer, like the one on a bolt. Those were the objects that sounded like his name I *mentally* stuck the rose into the washer and fixed this image on Mr. Rosenwasser's forehead. I've never forgotten his name, and since I see him maybe once every two years, he never fails to be amazed when I call him by name.

Sometimes, a name does not readily bring to mind an object that you can separately associate with the person's name. This was my problem when I met a fellow named, "Mears." Now, "Mears" is not an object, but it does sound like "tears." So, I immediately picture Mr. Mears with tears coming down his cheeks. Whenever I see him, I immediately see my mental picture of him crying and out comes Mr. (tears) Mears. Here are some other examples:

For the name of Fetterman, I thought of a tarred and feathered man. For Garbin, I thought of a tarpon (fish). For McCoy, I thought of the person holding a hillbilly rifle (the Hatfields and McCoys). Get the idea?

This skill for memorizing names can be developed to a fantastic degree and can come in mighty handy to salesmen, executives, teachers, or almost anyone.

But, you have to use your imagination with this system. The key is absurdity. Make the picture as "way out" as you can. You will better remember the person's name that way. The mind seems to remember the "unusual" better than the usual.

MEMORIZING THROUGH MNEMONICS

Do you know for certain which way to set your watch for day-light savings time? Do you know for certain when "I" comes before "E" in a word? How about the number of days in each month? These are the easy ones. Most everyone knows the sayings associated with them. But, how would you memorize the stops made by a street car in South Philadelphia? Or the color coding used on electrical resistors?

The principle is the same. It's done through mnemonics, which merely means a "*technique for remembering.*" (Did you look it up as per FLM #1?) Once you have mastered the technique of remembering mnemonically, you will come to feel that there is nothing worth remembering that doesn't have a mnemonic device to remember it by. And since memorizing is a big part of your education and studying, it's a good idea to learn the mnemonic way to memorizing. Here are some examples to show you how.

If you want to remember whether you move the hands of the clock forward or backward at those certain times of the year, just remember this mnemonic: "*Fall back and spring forward.*" That is, in the fall, move your clock back; in the spring move it forward.

If you want to remember whether a stalactite or a stalagmite hangs from the ceiling in a cave, just remember that the object has to be tight, as in stalactite, to hold on. The word stalagmite contains a "G" for ground. So, you will find stalactites hanging "tightly" from the ceiling and the stalagmite growing from the ground.

If you want to remember the names of the planets in the solar system, think of the sentence, "*My very earnest mother just served us nine pickles.*" The first letter of each word stands for the first letter of a planet and in the order they appear in the solar system. (*Mercury, Venus, Earth, Mars, Jupiter, Saturn, Uranus, Neptune, and Pluto.*)

Mario J. Giordano

Ask any electronic engineer how he remembers the color code on resistors and he will recite: "*Bad boys raped our young girls, but Violet gave willingly.*" The first letters stand for colors and their numerical values: 0 = black; 1 = brown; 2 = red; 3 = orange; 4 = yellow; 5 = green; 6 = blue; 7 = violet; 8 = grey; 9 = white"

In geography, a good way to remember the Great Lakes is to remember the word, "*homes.*" (Huron, Ontario, Michigan, Erie, and Superior.)

If you frequently ride a street car in South Philadelphia, you might recite this mnemonic to yourself: "*Red devils took my mother.*" (Reed Street; Dickinson Street; Tasker Street; Morris Street; Moore Street.)

If you want to remember the spelling of the word, "*Principal,*" think of the mnemonic, "*My pal is the principal*"

To spell the word, "*consul,*" think of "*Come out, Nina; see us laugh.*"

Physicians have to go through certain routines when they admit a patient to a hospital. If you ask one how he remembers the order of the routine, he will say, "*D.C. Van Dissel.*" (diagnosis, condition, vital signs, ambulatory, nursing orders, diet, intake and output, symptomatic drugs, special drugs, examinations, laboratory.)

Ask a biology student to list the Linnaean system of classification, and he will recite, "*King Peter came over from Germany seeking a fortune.*" (Kingdom, phylum, class, order, family, genus, species, form.)

I think I have given you enough examples to convince you that no matter what field, discipline, or career you're in, important data can be memorized mnemonically. All you need do is think up a catchy phrase or acronym that will represent items you're trying to remember.

It is amazing how simple this system is and how effectively it works in remembering even the most difficult things, like "pi" to the 14th decimal place. How about this mnemonic: "*How I want a drink, alcoholic of course, after the eight chapters involving quadric mechanics.*" (The number of letters in each word gives, 3.1415926535879," the value of "pi" to the 14th place.)

Now, very few people will have to remember "pi" to the 14th place, but if you are one of them, don't let it throw you. Just remember the mnemonic instead. It's easier and it never fails.

Mario J. Giordano

SOME LAST WORDS

You now have eight sure-fire, fast learning methods at your disposal. They are guaranteed to help you become a fast learner. Using any one of these eight methods can speed up the time it takes you to reach your goals.

By applying FLM #1 - The Three Golden Rules of Learning - you will remove the one major barrier to understanding. Your learning skills will take on the fineness of a well-constructed watch. At first, you may find yourself going to the dictionary quite often. Have the satisfaction of knowing that the more you use this FLM, the less - later on - you will need to.

By learning FLM #2 - A Fast Study Method That Guarantees High Test Scores - you'll make it almost impossible for you to fail any test. In fact, it will be difficult for you to make less than "A" in any course you take.

By applying FLM #3 - Speed Learning Through Individualized Instruction - you will master a method for learning any body of knowledge on your own, without the need for classes and teachers. By knowing about individualized instruction, you will never again have to tackle any job or course-of-study with fear of not knowing its technology.

By applying FLM #4 - Understanding Through Demonstrating With Objects - you will learn the way to restore to your education that which was most absent - the objects of your education. With simple bric-a-brac, you will bring "doingness" to your learning. You will "*lay in concrete*" what you attempt to learn.

By applying FLM #5 - Fast Learning By Selecting Out Data – you will learn how to zero in on the important facts of any body of knowledge. You will no longer be bothered in your studies with quantities of unimportant data.

By applying FLM #6 - Flash Reading For Understanding - you will learn the method of quickly absorbing the basics of any subject. It will give you a bedrock foundation to build on. No longer will you spend hours of reading. You'll flash scan a book to full understanding in a fraction of your average time.

By applying FLM #7 – Mini-Courses From Your Dictionary - you'll be able to get quick understanding at a moment's notice of the main data in any subject or about any job. It will show you how to quickly *close the loop* to understanding almost anything you want to know.

By applying FLM #8 - Tricks to Memorizing - never again will memorizing lists of data pose an impossible task for you. You'll learn how to memorize quickly and efficiently any data, and recall verbatim, even weeks later.

Any of these eight FLMs can be used as a "knowledge" way to achieve almost any goal. You have but to apply them to learn with certainty that when you increase your ability to learn, you also increase your chances to succeed.

ABOUT THE AUTHOR

Mario J. Giordano was an educator for 35 years; most of it at the college level. He graduated with honors with a B.S. in Education and an M.Ed. in Business Education from Temple University in Philadelphia. From the beginning of his career, he soon realized that the one thing schools didn't teach their students was *how to learn*! His expertise in education and business management lead him to create entire educational systems for the U.S. government and private industry. The methods described in this book were fundamental to the diffusion of educational information and have benefitted literally thousands of his students, including his own three sons. As a testimony to the efficacy of these methods, my younger brother, Gary, went from an unmotivated "C" student in high school to making the Dean's List in Junior College. He received a full scholarship from the United States Air Force to complete his B.S. at St. Joseph's University. After his military service, he returned to university, took some pre-requisite courses and was accepted to medical school. After graduation, he did his residency in Internal Medicine and passed his Board Examinations in the highest percentile. Today, he readily admits that he owes his success to our father for his methods of study. Prof. Giordano passed away in 1993 and never experienced the internet, but he would have been amazed and enthusiastic about how the dissemination of knowledge has been magnified and simplified.

Printed in Great Britain
by Amazon